Happiness Is a Way of Life

HAPPINESS
is a way of life

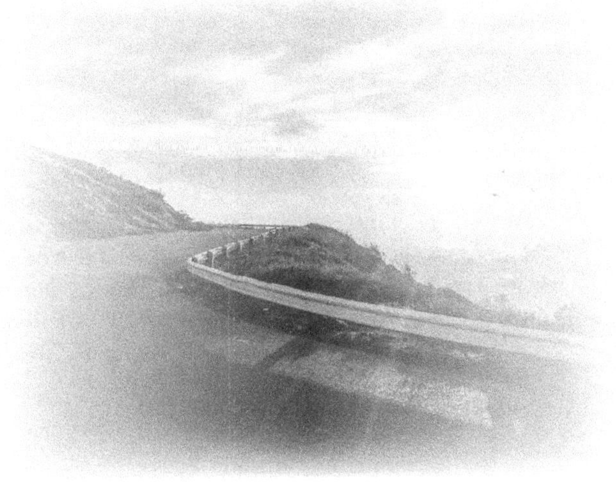

follow your path

J.H. Frenay

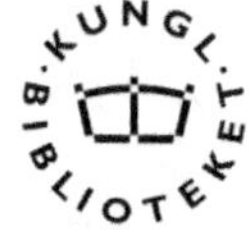

National Library
of Sweden

ISBN 978-91-527-7612-4 - Paperback
ISBN 978-91-527-7615-5 - eBook

Contents

Happiness is not in what we get.
Happiness lies in what we become.

— JIM ROHN

Introduction

The ideas and knowledge shared in the following pages have been learned, discovered and used along my own journey.

Whatever your beliefs or culture might be, this information is universal, and the way I've learned it is my own. Everyone has their own way of learning, sometimes similar, sometimes different.

It started when I was twenty. I asked myself and the universe: Who am I? Where do we come from? What is the purpose of life on Earth, and what is *my* purpose in life?

These questions, I carried for months and years, until step by step, I learned about spirituality, life and death, intuition and energy.

Some books came to me, written by people who shared their knowledge, and I also used my own intuition.

Through meditation and energy work, I found information and a connection to my higher self or soul.

One day my body finally reconnected to itself and to my soul.

How? I talked to it, directly and by looking at it in the mirror. I gave it love and the recognition that my body—everyone's body—is an amazing being, and each cell is a pure, beautiful conscious being that gives us the possibility to experience life. "No body, no life."

Our body is our temple

Literally, on Earth, through the body is how we experience everything. Meditate on that.

With the reconnection of my consciousness with my body, the connection to everything became clear and palpable.

It induced a feeling of being one with everything, which created a feeling of unconditional love.

We love what we relate to. How would you feel if you were one with everything? If all that exists were within you, and you were in all that exists?

You'd just love at an amazing level. At a level where judgement disappears and understanding appears.

This would be at a conscious level and an energetic level.

Then, the way to bring that consciousness into our daily life is through our thoughts, words, and actions.

Since I have reached this level of consciousness, I try to follow that consciousness and knowledge in my life. It is a challenge when you are alone and have a past that was not as easy as many of us have. At the same time, this consciousness of who we are and the purpose of life did help me get through the difficulties of daily life, emotional pain, and healing.

During the last twenty years, I experienced and learned more from that place of unity and connection than if I were not in that place at the time. The consciousness of who I am never left me, like riding a bike—once learned, it's forever.

I wish to share that experience with you today to help you on your own journey of discovery and the creation of your life and happiness. Through this book and via my spiritual coaching, energetical seance, guided meditation, and more, I will be honoured to be a stepping stone on your path.

Enjoy this book, enjoy your life, enjoy your body, and remember how beautiful you are.

CHAPTER 1

POWER OF PURPOSE

Reconnecting to Your Purpose and Goal

Why?

This is the question that will give us the most direct road to our goals, to our happiness, fulfilment, and wealth.

Did you ever think about why you do what you do? Why do you want to have kids, have this business, and want to be in a relationship with your friends, family, and lover?

Did you ever think about what makes you truly happy? And have you noticed when and what makes you happy? Whatever you want to improve, whether it is in your personal life, your business, or the society you live in, by answering those kinds of questions, you will grow more confidence, energy, happiness, fulfilment, and wealth in all areas of your life!

Why is it so important to know your goals and purpose in life?

It will give us the motivation to go forward every day. When you have a goal to reach, and you know the purpose of this goal, you feel alive and you feel connected to something you can achieve. You can see yourself grow in the process to get to your destination, and at the same time, you feel fulfilled by the road you take and by the lives you touch along this road.

Let me tell you one thing straight away. It will not be easy and pleasant all the time. Also, it will be great, and you will have fun and feel that you've accomplished something during the process of finding your goals and purpose.

What does it give us to know our goals and purpose?

Passion and life. Whatever your goal and purpose are, big or small, they will drive your thoughts. Your days will be filled up with more vigour, and you will have more energy than you ever had before when you know what you want. You'll accomplish something that really feeds your heart and soul and gives you the possibility to be wealthier in all areas of your life.

Take pen and paper and make a personal list of

questions. Start by writing down all that you do or want to do in your life. Then take your list and add a big WHY at the top, and for each thing you do or want, write an answer for why it is essential to you, why you do it or want to do it.

For some of your points, you might have nothing positive to say about it, and that is OK. Many people don't like their job but do it just for the money, for example. And when you find a point like that in your list, think about why it's not what you like or want—what is it giving you in the present moment?

A clear vision of what you want and don't want will help you take the best ACTION to make change, improve your life, and smooth out your path to a successful life. See the list of example goals below.

First, I have another point to share on this matter, and it starts with a question that I would like you to answer on a piece of paper before reading any further.

What do you do when you get good news or something good is happening in your life?

Most of us have the same answer: we share it, tell the people close to us, call our friends, or meet with the people we want to share the good news with.

Again, ask yourself, "Why?"

Because we are social animals. We love to connect, and for those who say, "Not me, I like to be alone," look how happy you are and how fulfilled your life is. Even if it's just with your family or your pet, you connect to feel alive.

A study showed that babies who were left alone all the time and just received the basic care, food, and a clean diaper let themselves die.[1]

That was a long time ago. Whatever we have in terms of material wealth, joyful times, or even painful times, it is never fulfilling if it is not shared. When you make your list of goals and purpose, constantly think about giving and sharing. Including yourself! Whatever you do, if it is more significant than just for yourself, you will feel happy and fulfilled, whatever it is you are doing!

List of example goals:
1. *I want to be or do (job, title)*
2. *I want to be or do an artistic profession, from actor to writer or even clarinet player.*
3. *I want to be a better father or mother for my kids.*
4. *I want to be an inventor.*

---

1. Frederick's Experiment: https://www.digma.com/digma-images/video-scripts/fredericks_experiment.pdf.

5. *I want to be a kinder person.*
6. *I want to be more connected with nature.*
7. *I want to be more connected with the people in my neighbourhood.*
8. *I want to be more openhearted.*
9. *I want to be more loved.*
10. *I want to be more listened to.*
11. *I want to be more compassionate.*
12. *I want to be more involved.*

Here's my own story of how having a goal gave me focus, determination, certainty, drive, and joy.

I was in the army for 15 years, and before leaving it, I was in a position where I did not like it anymore. From my situation and the conceptions I had about my personal life, I felt sad and depressed because I could not see a way out, which led me to burnout. I could not see where my life was going, and I did not want an unfulfilling job just to pay my bills and have no perspective in my life.

Through multiple events in the span of six months, I arrived at a point where all I had was gone: my 8-year-old son did not want to see me anymore, my girlfriend fell in love with someone else, and I lost my place to live after giving up my apartment to live together with that girlfriend.

And at this moment, when all was looking bad, what happened was actually the result of all my thoughts and desire to live a life more passionate, more fulfilling, more connected to my beliefs, soul, and heart.

My intuition or higher self, whatever you think it is, just pushed me hard and told me, "You go now," and I knew I had to travel, take a journey by foot for an undetermined length of time.

That's when one of my goals was born, and I did follow it. I took action directly by asking for a leave of absence without salary for a year, without knowing any details of my upcoming travel or how I would arrange my financial situation. I decided to first take action.

In the army, the administration can take a long time, and it eventually took four months to get the answer. But even without knowing if it would be yes or no, I just focused on my travel plans because I knew deep within me that it was my goal, and it was essential. Having this goal had put me in a state of unstoppable thriving. I was confident that I was going, so sure that I booked my train ticket four months before the date and before knowing the answer from the army. It made me feel happy, and I focused very firmly on my preparation and organization, from the material to the administrative points.

I had the chance to live with my sister for the months before I departed, and I arranged all my finances to be sure there wouldn't be any problems when I was gone. I paid off my loan at the bank, and one month before leaving, the balance on my account was zero. Neither positive nor negative. I was a happy man.

But because life always gives you what you need, I did get my last paycheck and my December bonus. I left at the beginning of December. And at that same time, when I had to call for the answer from the army, they sent me a yes.

All went well because when you touch your goal and even more, your purpose in life, and walk forward to reach it, life works *for* you and *with* you. This journey has been blissful, and I did learn and experience a lot in those eight months on the road. This book is a direct consequence of it.

I had a total of 16 months of holiday without an income, and in the end, I was left with less than 60 euros a month for the last nine months, but I never had to ask for food or anything else. All came to me.

Because of this journey, I quit the army and started a new life, first in the Netherlands and now here in Sweden. Finding a goal, focusing on it, and working to reach it leads us on a journey full of passion, full of adventure and challenges that make us grow and become wealthier inside and even materially too.

I realize this is a unique example, but it is an excellent way to see that without a purpose or a goal in life, we find it difficult to see where to go and how to feel happy, to thrive, and feel fulfilment.

I will finish this example by sharing the following with you.

All the wonderful and blissful moments I experienced during this journey happened when I shared or gave something to someone or to a being of any kind.

In mathematics, $1 + 1 = 2$, but in life, when someone shares their life, love, or passion with someone else, it is not just two persons who are touched but an exponential event that will connect way more people and create more energy than we can count or imagine. And this how we create the world the way we want to see it. We are more powerful than we could ever imagine.

This example was just about a goal, and OK, it was a big one for me. At the same time, I did not have a conscious purpose for this travel. I went into it as an open adventure without a plan.

In my early twenties, I discovered my deep purpose in life, and without really knowing how to achieve it, it has been a red line through every moment in my life since. Having my purpose in the background of my mind helped me get through difficult times.

Like during a four-year period when the frustration and anger that I'd suppressed for so long exploded and made my life difficult. My purpose gave me hope, courage, and something to look forward to when I was more often looking toward the darkness. To be reminded of my purpose by those who loved me when I could not see it has been a great asset to get me back on my feet and walking forward again in my life.

Having a purpose as your goal, whatever you want to achieve, gives you a greater feeling of accomplishment, of connection with yourself and all around you. It gives you a good sense of your power to create along the way. It makes you see that you can create the world you want to live in!

CHAPTER 2

POWER OF EMOTIONS

Let Them Own You
Or Own Them

Emotion, E-motion (energy in motion). For most of us, that is the force that drives us to act the way we do! I will come back to this later.

Emotions are the final results of our experiences of life. There is a connection between emotion, experience, and action, shown in the triangle diagram below. If we agree to start with our experiences, we understand that what we see, hear, and touch creates our understanding of the outside world through the filter of our body. All that information arrives inside our body and mind through a more sensitive filter, our brain (the analyzing part) and heart (the emotional part).

From those two receptive points, we start to feel some emotions, and we take actions directed by those emotions.

Those actions create new experiences, and the circle continues repeatedly.

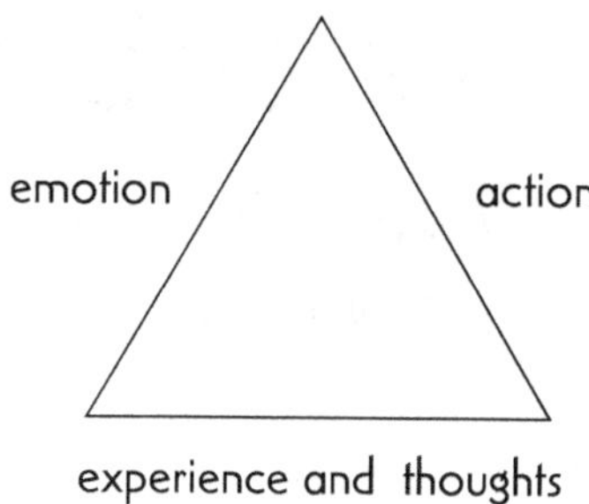

That is the basics of it, and it lays the groundwork for the chapter about the power of creation (Chapter 4), where we will go more into detail.

As we see in this triangle, emotions directly influence our experience of life and our way of dealing with the experiences that we live.

We can define emotions as positive and negative even if we know that positive and negative emotions don't actually exist. What we do have are emotions that help you to reach what you desire and those that put you far away from the results you are after.

The emotion is alive only inside you, and only you

can give it a colour, a purpose, and a level of importance in your life.

When positive emotions control you, like joy for example, it's not much of a problem. When we feel joy, we might make some stupid mistakes under the euphoria of the moment, but nothing harmful happens most of the time.

When it is an emotion like anger or jealousy, this can be more destructive. My experience living in anger for almost four years showed me this was ugly.

I let this emotion make me do hard things to the person I love the most. I screamed. I used foul language and hurtful words. I showed physical signs of aggression (without acting on it), making me feel horrible inside. I hurt people, and at the same time, being angry hurt me a great deal too, emotionally and physically.

The effect of emotions on our physical body

This point is essential: all emotions create a chemical reaction in our body. It is a chain reaction of electric influx, a production of different hormones and chemical substances that make our body react. Depending on the body's emotion, the reaction chain will proceed in a specific pattern. Happiness is hugely different from anger, and unconditional love is also very different from hate.

The emotions that come from experiences that create more life, love, and fulfilment will have a different impact on the body than those that come from emotions that create fear, disconnection, and sadness.

"Motion creates emotion."
— Tony Robbins.

As our friend Tony Robbins said in his decades of work, movement is an efficient tool to change your emotions. It will not stop you from being affected by them, but it will help you transform one emotion into another.

If you don't like what you feel because that doesn't bring you where you want to be, you can try to change it into an emotion that will more likely get you where you want to be, and movement is an excellent way to do so.

Putting your body in a position that makes you feel the emotion you wish to feel, or even smiling mechanically, will make you happier, because the brain doesn't know the difference. Breathing more deeply will also help.

Let us make a little exercise list to help to change your emotions.

Stand up straight, with your head up and shoulders low and back, opening your chest. If you feel depressed, put a smile on your face, and "fake it till you make it."

Our brain will not see the difference because it can't distinguish between what we experience or imagine. Studies show that if we eat an apple or only imagine eating an apple, the same place in the brain reacts in the same way. I repeat for the smart ones: You have to do it, not just imagine it!

Go play a sport, go for a walk, dance, laugh out loud, play with your kids, do something crazy, whatever it takes. Change what you are doing when you want to change how you feel. The world of emotion is massive, and I don't want to write a whole book about it. It simply comes down to the core of it, seeing what emotions really are.

Our emotions get created by our life experiences, from when we were born until our deaths. They are only one part of us. When we are born, we are already complete, which means that the world of emotion inside of us is not who we are. The ego is a part of this world of emotions, and what we think of as our personality is a mix of emotions and our true selves.

The true self is the part of you that can think outside of the emotion. It is the one who asks inside yourself, "Why do I feel sad?" If you can see that you are a conscious being who thinks and can act consciously, independently of the emotion you feel, you have gained an idea of the world of emotion and your power within it.

In this stage, you can stop identifying yourself with your feelings. You will not say, "I am sad," you will instead say, "I feel sadness within me." This distinction can open a new way for you to start dealing more positively and efficiently with your world of emotions and regain confidence and control of your life.

Look at the world of your emotions from a further distance. It looks like a cloud full of little hands trying to pull you in. When you let yourself fall back into the shadow of your emotions, you are in its midst and you cannot see clearly what is happening. Then, you make decisions based on the emotions that block your inner vision, and the results are not the best you could have.

Do this exercise: whatever emotion you feel, look at it from an outside perspective, putting yourself in the position of an observer, with no judgment and no labels on the feeling. Sadness or happiness is not bad or good. It is just sadness or happiness, like blue and black are neither good nor bad.

When you can observe your emotions without judgment, you will be more able to come back to the state of an observer when necessary. The goal here is not to dispose of all emotions, but to become the master of their powers; it is possible! Being the observer will allow you to feel your inner voice, intuition, or higher self, depending on what you call it. It will guide you with a greater purpose. It will always bring you to the path that gives more and creates more life and abundance, not only for you but for all. This is the path that puts all your choices through the lens of unity—the understanding that we are all one.

Emotion is the force that drives us to act the way we do. For most of us! Why for most of us? Because some rare people on this planet have learned and mastered the world of emotions, and are not owned by them but use them as a tool, or just see them without really interfering with them.

Those people have achieved significant work on their self-control and discipline through meditation, ritual, and exercises like the one explained earlier. They manage to stay in a state of happiness most of the time and don't let unwanted emotions drive them. If they observe an emotion that creates a different result than the one they're after, those people directly take action to change them and get back into a state that procures them what they want to feel, experience, and create.

You can observe some of the wealthiest (in all aspects of their life) people in this world living their life happily and healthily, no matter whatever happens in their life.

The gift of criticism

How can we see a gift in the criticism of others? There is an excellent side to receiving the critiques of others. Positive or negative, when a person gives us criticism, they express their personal opinion formed through their own paradigm, knowledge, and beliefs.

To be honest, we don't care about that. We don't judge the person who critiques us; we send them love! What is particularly important here is, what do you feel when you receive criticism? There lies the gift of criticism.

We need to be quick at this game. Our awareness of what we feel needs to be sharp. If you can directly feel and recognize the feeling you have when you receive criticism, ask yourself this question:

What does this touch in me?

For example, somebody criticizes your way of doing something, and you realize it makes you feel insecure. If you don't think about it, you may go on the defence and answer with some aggression in your voice.

But if you understand that whatever is said to you is not about you but about what the other person is experiencing, you are free to focus on your feelings and ask yourself, why do you feel insecure at this comment?

The answer can be that you don't feel good enough and don't have high confidence in yourself. Then you open the door to receiving the gift of criticism. You may learn that you have to do something about your self-confidence or knowledge of other aspects of yourself!

It is essential to recognize the critique not as a judgment but as an opportunity to grow, not by what is said to you but by the way it makes you feel. In the same way, it will also open your mind and heart to receive criticism that can be constructive and helpful. Though you may feel bad about what's said to you, it may be something that you have to hear.

My friend and neighbour told me a long time ago, Jean, you handle your son like he is in the military, but you are softer with your stepchildren. It hurt me and made me cry because I could accept the truth in it, and by making no defence but accepting the gift of criticism, I was able to start the process of being less strict and being softer on my son.

Letting go!

Wow! Easier said than done! Letting go: it's an easy saying which often comes to you when you worry, or through some healing therapies, or from psychologists, but they never tell you how to do that.

Let me tell you, to let go is not easy and straightforward; it's a process where you transform what you don't want anymore and replace it with what you desire, with a new and better understanding.

I will give you an example. When you lose someone dear to you and keep grieving, people tell you, "Let it go, go on with your life." But how do you do that?

Acceptance of the situation is one of the keys, to begin with. The second is trying to understand the situation and how you can make it positive. Don't try to suppress what happened and forget all about it. That's not possible. But at the same time, please don't put all your time and attention into it. Live your life as usual, or even better, in a new, more positive way than before. Give the loss of your dear one a meaning for you to live a better life.

That is just one example, and it will be different for other situations. One common point is that what you focus on sticks and grows. The more you focus on what you want to let go of, the more it will stick around. You know it's there, but you give your focus to something else, to the opposite maybe, or to some other constructive activity.

Focusing blindly on your job or sport or some other thing will just push away the problem for a while, and it will come back stronger. Give some deep thought to what you want to let go of and then act upon it. Don't try to avoid it!

For some people, this will come fast as they understand some of these principles, and for others, it will take a long time until a new understanding takes place.

Don't beat yourself up, be gentle with yourself and go forward in all your activities, and you will get there. You will let go of what is blocking you and look back on it as a bad dream without even noticing it.

It all depends on the right moment for you—you cannot run before you learn to walk!

CHAPTER 3

POWER OF INTUITION

Our Inner Compass

Intuition—what is it?

We call it many names: our gut feeling, the little voice in our head, or as my father called it, the hair under his feet.

It's a feeling deep inside that sounds or feels right, a sense of certainty about something you don't know in advance. Your ability to know the way you have to take, even if reason tells you no, and wants you to take the familiar way as always.

When you start to notice your intuition, don't judge it, don't kill it directly with mental analysis. Instead, act on it. It is scary initially, because your intuition can ask you to do something you're not familiar with or take a way that is the opposite of your belief system. When you start to listen to it, it will become sharper.

Intuition works for everything in your daily life, at home or at your job. Many of us have experienced this when driving without really looking where we're going. How many drivers have been alerted intuitively that we should slow down for no apparent reason, when boom, a car appears out of nowhere, or the one in front of us brakes abruptly?

When I was in the army, I had an intuition about a problem we were having with a truck, and when I went to check it, bingo! It was exactly what my intuition had told me, without even checking anything else.

Following your intuition can become a life changer when taken to a higher level of consciousness and practice.

In my own life, I experienced it to this level. When I was travelling by foot for eight months, I was free of concern about anything. I was free to follow my intuition without fear of getting lost or attacked or anything else. That intuition became my first guide, most of the time before my mind. When I set a point to go to, my intuition would guide me there, and it brought me what I needed.

For example, when it was almost my birthday, I

told myself that I wanted to be in a good place with pleasant people and have a wonderful birthday. That was two days before my birthday. The following day, my intuition told me to go hitchhiking, even though I had committed to just walking to Lisbon, a hundred kilometres further.

But I listened, I lifted my thumb up, and in no time, a truck pulled over and brought me close to Lisbon. For the remaining distance, I took a local bus and arrived in the city centre. There I searched for a good and cheap place to sleep, since my finances at this time were still small.

My intuition again made me notice a beautiful woman at the hostel entrance. I went there and found the place was beautiful, cheap, and the people were very friendly.

The next day I took action to make this day special. It was my birthday, after all. I gave free hugs in the street, and like that, I met four Italian women who wanted a free hug. We talked, and after a moment, they invited me to spend the rest of the afternoon with them and to have dinner with them that night. It was a perfect birthday present, and I even got a little chocolate cake with a candle on it to blow out.

Following my intuition so trustingly made me wonder who was in charge, because I felt like I was no longer in charge. My intuition became like an outside thought that was not attached to me. It was like I got the information from outside of my head. And that is indeed the case.

Your intuition is your cells resonating with your goals and objectives, and it will give you the feeling that you are on the right path to achieving what you desire, or arriving where you want to be. At the same time, it is a knowledge greater than yourself. It will tell you what you need to focus on the most and the least, to achieve what you want in your mind. Intuition resonates with your most profound purpose and goals, and with what you keep alive in your heart, even if you are not conscious of it.

To understand more about intuition and its importance, we have to look at who we are as human beings.

Independently of our culture and beliefs, we need to look at the core of our being: ENERGY!

Scientists from all places, cultures, and religions agree that through the latest research in quantum physics, all matter is energy expressing itself in different frequency waves.

We are conscious energy beings, and our vibration gets to a level where we become matter—the body. The trick is that we are not just the body, energy goes everywhere, and we are not limited in space. We certainly become more ether, less compact in our energy field as it goes further and further, and still, we are bound to this energy.

The most significant thing is that it is conscious energy. We can tap into the unlimited field of information that all beings and the universe contain by understanding this.

It is where our intuition goes and takes the information it gives us—the field of energy around us!

Using intuition to its full potential

We have different uses for our intuition at various levels.

We have the basic use for our daily life. For example, a mother who feels something is happening with her kids playing in their room.

This intuition is the one that we can learn to follow, even if sometimes we make a mistake. By trusting more in the feeling, it will become clearer and more present in our life. Pay attention to your little voice.

The second use is for a bigger purpose, our conscious goals and purpose. In the same way, we have to be present and give our attention to the signs and the feelings we get. Life gives us a tremendous amount of information and guidance throughout our process. But by being so busy, entertained and distracted, we cannot hear it, feel it, or see it.

Watch less television and play video games less, take some time to just rest in silence, and feel yourself breathing in and out. This is an excellent exercise to calm the mind and start to feel and hear your inner voice. In this case, intuition gives us some feelings and knowledge. Also, it provides us with external signs to guide us. Again, we have to trust it, and in the beginning, we may take our thoughts for intuition and make mistakes. The more you practice trusting your gut, the more it becomes effective.

The third use is the more unconscious one, as our intuition helps us at a deep level to give us what we need to grow and be more fulfilled.

How and why?

How? By giving us thoughts, feelings, and events in our life that don't make sense at first or scare us. But if we can take in those events or persons and ideas, then we can grow, solve some serious problems, breakthrough some old patterns, and open a new page of our experience.

This type of intuition is the most difficult to see and

accept because it needs us to be aware of the changes we need to make.

Why? Because we are conscious beings and alive. Life always supports life. If a system or an organism doesn't follow the laws of nature and life, it will disappear.

Life will always thrive, and in this same way, we are here to grow and always be a better and greater expression of life. That is why we feel pushed to be more alive, whether we want it or not. This hunger for life makes us feel uncomfortable, sad, or bad when we go against it.

By going back to following our inner senses, our intuition, we will be able to go with the flow of life and grow in all aspects of life—relations, work, money, our self-consciousness, happiness, and our sense of being more than just what we do, of being alive and part of something way more significant than just ourselves. We are a part of an ecosystem called the universe!

Connect to your intuition

Here's an exercise to connect to your intuition and tap into the universal library.

We first have to understand why we get disconnected from our intuition. As I said before, we are way too distracted by all the entertainment around us. Television, radio, video games—the information we get from everywhere is negative, ninety-nine percent of the time. It puts us into a state of worry and takes our calm and focus away. We have all the unimportant chit-chats during the day because we have lost the confidence to speak our minds and be honest.

All of those things and more take our energy and mind to a space where there is always noise. When was the last time you were in a quiet place with just yourself, doing nothing? No smartphone or computer, no TV, nobody else—just you and the silence.

To start, we have to make time for ourselves, even if it's just ten minutes to start with in the beginning.

Be quiet with no distractions at all. And just breathe, focus on the feeling of the air passing through your nostrils, in and out. This exercise will help you calm down the noise of your thoughts, and the more you practice, the more you will be able to focus for a long time before the flow of your thoughts interferes. Just come back to the feeling of the air every time you drift away in your mind.

Use it every time you can, while waiting at a red light in traffic, or when you're eating. Feel your body, scan it part by part and just observe what you feel at each place, and then move to another part of it.

And very importantly, be quiet whenever you can. Don't speak about just anything, learn to talk about what is essential and not just make noise. If you want to grow your intuition, the first step is being focused on those exercises. And every time you can, practice silence, and during the silence, you can practice the breathing technique and focus on your body.

Then listen to what comes to you: feelings, ideas, images, or events, the need to go somewhere or speak to a certain person, someone you know or not.

I had an experience during my travel, in the cathedral of Santiago de Compostella, at the end of the pilgrimage route that carries the same name, when I felt attracted by three people talking together. I followed my intuition, which told me to speak to the youngest of the women.

After a brief introduction and talk with her and her parents, I asked if I could visit her when I passed through the village where she lived, where I planned to go a few days later. She said yes and gave me her phone number.

I met her there three days later, and long story short, we had two beautiful days together. I gave her some energy therapy too. She acknowledged that she was scared at first and usually would never meet with someone that she didn't know, but she accepted because she dreamed about me the night before seeing me in Santiago and recognized me.

Consciously or not, we are guided through all aspects of our lives and the lives of others. We are interconnected. Finally, on this point, judgment is a big key to not failing, not only for your intuition but for everything. Learn to stop any kind of judgment about yourself or others, about what is good or not. Learn to look at your thoughts, and when you see a judgment, stop it, say no, and think a positive thought to replace your judgment. Find a pleasant thing to say about what you were judging, even if it's a small thing.

In the beginning, it's arduous work; you brainwash yourself because we have so many ways to judge ourselves, and we've done that since we were very young.

When you catch a judgmental thought, do something that will make you react—speak loudly, or like I used to do, pinch yourself. The physical pain reminded me of the pain that judgmental thought causes to my body and life.

Judgment takes a lot of space, time, and energy from our life. By reducing it, we have more room to have the thoughts that we want. Then the information that we receive all the time has more space to go through the flow of the mind.

Intuition is like the compass of the character

Jack Sparrow in *Pirates of Caribbean.* It will show you the direction of the thought you hold the most. If you change all the time, the compass will change direction too, but when you focus, it will point in the same direction.

CHAPTER 4

POWER OF CREATION

What really is the law of attraction, and how can we use it?

Good news for all of us. We already do it all the time.

First, we have to put the base of it with the question, "Who are we?"

I will invite you to do a little exercise before reading further. Close your eyes and ask yourself this question, "Who am I?"

Let it sink in, don't search. It's best to do this every day until an answer comes to you. Of course, I do understand your desire to read further.

Here is my answer:

To put it briefly, Antoine Lavoisier said, "Nothing is lost, nothing is created, everything is transformed."

And Einstein said: "Energy cannot be created or destroyed, it can only be changed from one form to another."

ENERGY! Conscious energy, simply, is what we are. But let's take this a bit deeper to allow everyone to understand this concept.

We are tripartite beings; we have our body, mind, and spiritual being (also called our soul: our conscious energy.)

If we look deeper or expand our point of view, we can see that those three parts are the same thing in different forms: energy.

Energy is everywhere and in everything. Quantum physics has determined that at the smallest state, matter becomes a wave. All around us, the matter we see is made of moving atoms and electrons. Those electrons and atoms are themselves made of the tiniest particles, and then it becomes a wave—energy!

I believe that we humans are made of energy which is pushed by a conscious power known as life force, chi, or spiritual consciousness.

Our core is one of intelligence and conscious energy that takes different states of vibration to create matter, our body, and our mind. By understanding this, we will close the gap of our false belief in the separation between ourselves and whatever we want to create, and then we can attract it toward ourselves.

Imagine everything around you like a radio station: your fridge is channel one, your television is channel two, and your dream job is channel three. How can you attract the thing you want in your life?

Tune yourself to the right channel and stay focused on it as long as is necessary to manifest it in your life.

Now comes the critical point: how do I tune myself to the one thing I desire in my life?

Think, think, think, and think again.

Feel, feel, feel, and feel again.

Then take action, take action, take action and take action again.

And repeat.

Thinking is something we do all the time, and most of it, we do not control. We get overrun by a train of useless thoughts, and in a lot of cases, it makes us feel anxious or worried. We have to learn to take control of our thoughts.

Energy waves

Thoughts are manifested in our brain and body by an electrical exchange in the brain. Our energy waves show evidence of why we have to take control of our thoughts. Every thought is a wave, and it attracts and tunes itself in to the same energy wave.

By making our mind quieter, or at least being more focused and not letting our train of thought disturb the thoughts we consciously create, we can stay focused and tune in to what we desire to create for a more extended period.

One of the best ways to train your mind is to remember that the train of thought running in your mind is not you.

Let me show you a simple exercise.

You certainly have been in a situation where you were scared or stressed. At that time, a lot of thoughts were going on, but for one moment you said to yourself, "OK, OK, calm down. It's OK…"

If you can, recall this moment, or the next time it happens to you, take a moment to ask if you can think about being calmer when your mind is running crazy. What does that mean? Who is really in charge? Who is saying, "OK, OK, calm down. It's OK…"?

You are in charge, but it's better to come to realize this by yourself, by training yourself to observe your train of thought.

You are the observer

We lose our power as co-creators and observers by unconsciously thinking that our thoughts are who we are!

But there's good news! With a bit of practice and determination, you can train yourself to be less and less affected by the thoughts you don't choose and instead create and focus on the thoughts you choose to have.

First, remember that you are the observer of the thoughts, not the thoughts themselves! Repeat it again and again, write it on a piece of paper that you carry with you, and use it every time you can.

Meditation is a perfect way to grow your skills as an observer. Use the technique of feeling the air going in and out through your nostrils. By focusing on a physical aspect, you give a job to your mind, which is not yet able to let the train of thought go out of the station. The mind will win a lot in the beginning, but the more you practice, the more you will be in control and make your mind focus.

Don't judge yourself; it takes time and a lot of practice. Try one hour a day, or every stop at a red traffic light. When you are committed to it, I will advise you to visit a retreat to practice Vipassana (a type of meditation that focuses on the body). There are Vipassana centres worldwide, and they are based on donations, so your budget will never be an obstacle.

Doing this will give you an excellent start, and it will be easier to continue at home, plus you will gain all the other benefits that come with this retreat.

Another exercise is to go on a walk every morning, talk aloud to yourself, express in words what you are grateful for, then set some goals and objectives for the day or week, and finish with some good affirmations about yourself.

At the same time, use this to work on yourself, or to find answers for a problem you may have in your life. When you talk to yourself out loud, you are active, you are in command of what you say, and because you think about what you want to say, your mind cannot interfere with your conscious discussion.

Be active in your thinking; when you let the train of thought go, it goes everywhere and nowhere. Be active, ask good questions that may require positive and constructive answers. Ask good questions, and then good answers and good thoughts will come.

The more work you give to your mind, the less your useless train of thought can leave the station. But be careful; all the entertainment that makes you brain-dead—focusing on a movie or game, or alcohol, or whatever—is not a positive and constructive way to stop the train of thought. To grow and to catch the prize you desire, you need to get up and work for it, and working on yourself can be one of the longest and most demanding jobs, one that's never really done. But the results are amazing!

Feel, feel, feel, and feel again.

Whatever the level of control over your thoughts, when you want to create something, you need to think and imagine your goal, make it into an image in your mind. When you have a good picture of the goal you're after, take it to the emotional level. Use all your imagination to create a movie inside your mind, bring the future into your present self.

Imagine living in the home you dream of; imagine being with your child the way you want and not how you used to be. Imagine yourself doing the job you really want to do.

By doing so, your brain will be directly in the same state as if you were actually doing your dream job or living in your dream house. The brain doesn't see the difference between material experience and dream experience.

For example, we all have been worried about

someone who we were waiting on to return from a party or someone who was going on a trip. Because we did not receive news fast enough or they were later than expected, we may have started to play a stupid, catastrophic movie in our head that made us feel bad.

If you follow me, you know what I mean by our brains not seeing any difference between reality and imagination.

Here's another important connection. Emotion comes from the ideas and concepts we have. Our thoughts become emotions, and where do we feel emotions?

It depends on which emotion! Love is felt in the heart, but anger goes to your stomach and liver. Like they say in the movie *Eat, Pray, Love,* you must smile "even with your liver!"

Here, we will focus on the heart for all emotions.

The heart is an organ with an autopilot. In the foetus, the heart starts to beat before the brain's formation.

Studies show that the heart sends more information to the brain than the brain sends to the heart.

In my research for this book, I found studies that showed the heart has its own intrinsic nervous system that consists of about 40,000 neurons that can send information to the brain. These neurons may play a role in memory transfer and emotion. The heart also communicates with the brain through hormones, pressure waves and electromagnetic fields.

What is most important for us to know here is that the magnetic field of the heart is 5,000 times stronger than the one in the brain. The magnetic field of the heart extends four meters around the body.

At the same time, the energy that it sends all around us goes way further than that. It doesn't have limits. Instead, it's a wave that goes through everything and everywhere.

That is a significant point for us to understand. When you want to create, you have to feel it, feel the emotions that come with the fulfilment of your goal. When you can feel that in your heart, the wave is sent out at an infinite speed all around you, and then on the way it hits the same wave, and connections are made.

You are not aware of it yet, but it is there, and if you can stay focused (tuned) on this wave, emotions are created by the image you imagined. You will send messages and receive messages and attract the experience of your thoughts.

Here, I advise you to reread the chapter about intuition! Your intuition will guide you to the objective, and intuition is the path revealed in front of you. You also see the way by asking a good question, and then a good thought will come with a good feeling around it.

Take action, take action, take action, and take action again

OK, if you made it until this point, that's good, but it will mean nothing if you don't follow the message you are receiving. Here is the real deal for changing your life, getting what you desire, and creating it in your mind and heart.

Taking action can be the most difficult part for some of us. It asks us to go past the line of fear, crossing the border of our comfort zone. At the same time, it is the ultimate way to get what we seek.

We have different ways to take action without being blocked by our fear and doubt.

Speed! You feel it, and you have the intuition to do it. You've thought about it, and you know it's what you need to do to get there.

Go, do it fast, jump, take action on it now, and then when you cannot go back, you will have time to shit your pants! And at the same time, you will feel some euphoria from being somewhere you've never been, out of your comfort zone.

Finding yourself with your back against the wall is also the time when you need to go and take action, even if you are afraid. When your situation can't get worse, and when life shows you the way to get through it, it puts you in a position where the only way is up, even if it's scary!

You can also ask for help from another person to boost your confidence, to give you support and rules, and just be a positive support. They may give you some kicks in the butt if necessary, but always with love.

Have courage and strength. You can see your fear and your doubt, but you do it anyway because you love yourself and your family and the community you live in, even the entire world. You know that by giving the best of you to the world and to yourself, you give the gift that you chose to be when you came into this world.

CHAPTER 5

POWER OF FOCUS AND DETERMINATION

Now that we've covered who we are and some parts about energy, we can start to see how essential focus and determination are.

The question now is what to focus on to create a happier, more fulfilled, joyful, and richer life in all aspects.

The first thing will be what you desire. The relationship, the new car, the quality time and interactions with your kids or yourself. It can be anything inside of you or outside!

This is and could be the only thing we focus on. You may have heard this quote from Tony Robbins:

Where focus goes, energy flows.

Because your focus is on putting all of your thoughts in one direction and sending it all around you, the energy of these thoughts is what you desire. Then the universe takes these thoughts and collects all of the same energy, sends it toward you, and makes you go out to find it.

Focusing is not only putting all your thoughts on one thing, but also increasing their power, like a laser is a concentrated light focusing on one place.

Every thought you have during the day needs to be turned towards the direction of your desire, whatever you are doing, because you are "all in one." You need to give the same focus to your thoughts about your goal as you do your thoughts about being a father or a wife or a football player.

I think if you've come this far in this book, you're one of those people who have the desire to grow in their life. What we've learned is that if we want to be happy in our lives and have a sense of fulfilment, then we need all aspects of our lives to give us the same joy and desire.

We can feel fulfilled in a job or feel fulfilled financially but still have poor relationships. And having fulfilling relationships may not be the thing that makes us feel fulfilled in our career or as a mother.

Now our determination comes into the game. How committed are we to pursuing our happiness and goals?

We need to commit and create a way to have determination and focus. Again, it comes with an idea and a feeling. We need to feel a push inside or from the outside. From the outside is easy! Being at the bottom of the pit means the only way to go is up, which gives us the motivation and determination to focus on our goals, behaviours, and thoughts!

The second way is to feel a push from the inside. We create a new idea by ourselves, and we want to become this new idea of ourselves. We want to be kinder, stronger, wealthier, but it's not just like the million people that say that every day from an empty heart. No, it's when you really see, think, and feel deep in your heart this new 'you' that the determination emerges, and you can focus more easily.

To find the determination within you without having to chase it, as we all have done at one point, we need to approach it from the perspective of what we want to *be* and not what we want to *have*.

Let me explain this clearly with this example.

We want to be wealthy, or we want to be rich. What is the difference?

Being rich means having lots of money and possessions. It's something that can change at any time. If you succeed at becoming rich, it can always disappear the following day.

Being wealthy is a state of being. When we feel wealthy, nothing can take it away, and as you now know, what we feel the most, we attract. And the benefits of feeling wealthy aren't limited to the material life—we can feel wealthy about our relationships, friendships, health, spirituality, and all other aspects of our life.

By feeling wealthy inside, if you lose all your possessions, you can still feel wealthy about the other aspects of your life, and this goes for anything you decide to attach to it. Feeling wealthy will bring you wealth in all aspects of your life.

This is where we all want to be, feeling good, happy, and fulfilled. This book and thousands of others are all about what we want to feel, and not what we want to have. When we search for new possessions, a relationship, a friend, or an extreme sport, we do so to experience greater feelings, to be alive, happy, and fulfilled.

Right there is the purpose of all of our actions. It's why we have to focus on one crucial element— the heart—where we feel, connect, and send to the world the energy that will attract into our physical life what we focus on.

We need to work with the conscious mind and the unconscious mind. We need to solve the issues of our past and grow as the person we are now, and we need to work and focus on our heart—the physical one, and the energetical one.

To do so, we need to realize that it's in the heart that we create everything in our life. The latest studies on the heart show that the state of it influences our mind, our mood, and our health. We are so interconnected inside and outside our body-mind.

How to focus on the heart and make it the best co-creator and friend you ever had?

The fastest and most efficient way is through unconditional love, kindness, and honesty! Those words are key in this process.

We have to remember that we are all good, that we are all connected, and we need to tear down all of the differences and walls between us. We are one race on earth, the human being, and we are one ecosystem on earth—nature, animals, and humans! Energetically we are not separated. The illusion of separation is that we have the conscious perception of being ourselves in one place, and that other beings are themselves somewhere else. Molecules of water are all unique, from the water molecules in the seas, oceans, rivers, and even the water in the atmosphere. All water around the world is connected. If it looks like the water is cut off and isolated from the oceans, the water in the air still connects all of the water molecules on earth, even in our bodies. Our energy connects us all.

Our heart directs a lot more in our body and life than we can imagine. You might know several sayings about the heart such as, "follow your heart," or "put your heart into it," and not without reason. These sayings transcend cultural and linguistic boundaries. In art, most people are touched by a sculpture, painting, or music because the artist did their work with imagination and feeling, and not just with excellent technique. They put their heart into it, and we can see and feel it.

The heart gives meaning to life.

To work on coming back to the heart, we can use meditation, affirmation, and gratitude. We can use energy and lithotherapy for example.

Let me give you an exercise to connect and open your heart.

First, the physical heart. Sit and put yourself in a calm state by using the breathing exercise I mentioned earlier. Now focus on feeling the pulse of your heartbeat in your body wherever you can. Then, try to focus on the heart itself. Feel it beating. Put your index and middle finger together, straighten them, and with the tips of your fingers touch your heart and let your fingers rest there.

As you feel your heart for as long as you're able, become the beat of your heart, and listen to what it can tell you about yourself and your body. Follow your intuition to go further in this process.

The second thing you can do (or just do this exercise on its own if you like) is touch your heart like I explained in the first exercise and then close your eyes to focus on your heart.

Imagine inside your heart one candlelight, while breathing in and out deeply. Try to intensify the light, not growing it in size directly but making it brighter.

In doing so, when you inhale, the light becomes brighter. When you feel that you can do so, make it grow when you exhale, too.

At first, make it grow for yourself inside your heart and body. Breathe in, and the light gets brighter; breathe out and the light goes further inside your heart and body. Imagine that all the shadows in all the corners of yourself are filling with light.

Don't force yourself—you will discover more in yourself than you could imagine. Don't judge. Just let the light be everywhere. Then make it grow around you. Again, breathe in, and the light is brighter, and out, and the light grows further.

Do it until you expand the light as far as you can, to your loved ones, your village and city, your country, the world, and beyond. Imagine the light touching everyone, every plant and animal, all elements on earth and further on. Feel connected, feel yourself being one with all.

What works well is to look at yourself in the mirror and focus on your heart. Imagine a bridge of light or a rainbow coming from your own heart into the reflection of your heart in the mirror. Tell your mirror image how beautiful you are, tell your mirror image, "I love you," and tell it, 'I am kind, I am one, I am light.'

Use whatever words you desire, but choose them carefully because the words you put in your heart affect you and everything in your life. Focus on the beautiful being you are and recognize it in more ways than you have ever done before. Judgment cannot be a part of this work if you truly desire to open your heart to create a better life for yourself and others!

What is essential to focus on?

To be able to develop ourselves in all aspects, we need to focus on the body and what we feel from it, as well as the information it gives us. It can tell us about our health, and it gives us the sensations that come with the experiences we have every day.

To provide a clear example, remember that when you get stressed, you feel warm, your heartbeat goes faster, your palms grow damp, and you might shake.

For every emotion you feel, you have biological activity that you can feel and focus on. By recognizing those reactions, you will be able to act consciously, making choices before you let your old patterns and reactions begin.

The second thing to focus on is your mind, your thoughts. And among those thoughts, two are a priority for me: judgement and self-love.

Judgment, because we have grown up in an environment where everything is judged and measured by everyone!

By focusing on our thoughts and judgments about others, about ourselves and everything else, we'll be able to see what is behind our judgments and we will be able to reconnect with the world and the people around us.

Every time you catch yourself judging, change the judgment to something positive. You have to find the positive in the person, the situation, or the thing you are judging. There is always something positive to see.

By doing so, you will not only stop judging, but you will also create a pattern of positivity that will make you see all the positive possibilities and qualities in everything you focus on.

It is a difficult job because we are so unconscious of all the little comments we have in our mind about everyone and everything, and even if we practice for a long time, we still have some judgment toward ourselves and others without wanting it.

It's worth doing!

Focusing on self-love and self-esteem is a key to happiness. Give yourself the love and recognition you seek from outside yourself. Tell yourself what an amazing person you are, what a beautiful spiritual being you are. Identify your good qualities and abilities, and tell them to yourself in the mirror. Believe sincerely that you are more than you think, or than what people say to you. Be kind to yourself.

One other point and important concept is where to focus. I learned that when you don't want something and you want to change it, most people focus on that: "I don't want *that* in my life, I want to change it." And they spend ninety percent of their time thinking that and only ten percent searching for a solution.

Whatever it may be, spend a minimum of time recognizing and having a clear vision of what you want to change—what you don't want any more, problems in your job or relationships—and then forget it.

Then, spend all your remaining time creating something that will make the thing you don't want obsolete, or finding a solution to your problem. Stop speaking about the issue, just speak about the possible solutions, because again, where focus goes, energy goes.

I can focus on the fact that I fall on the ground and stay there, saying it and complaining, but that will not make me stand up.

CHAPTER 6

RELATIONS AND FAMILY

Who You Stick With, You Become

You'll hear this in all of the courses, seminars, or other conferences from high achievers: *Who you stick with, you become!*

Why? It's simple: energy and example.

First, energy.

As we've seen before, everyone is comprised of energy, and this energy is represented as a wave in quantum physics. Studies show that every object, including the organs of our body and the body in its totality, have specific wave frequencies. And by taking as an example one apple and introducing this apple to a different frequency, the result is the modification of the frequency of the apple.

We know that all of our thoughts have unique frequencies, and a group of thoughts makes a pattern for our behaviour. And vice versa. Our behaviour creates and reinforces those patterns and groups of thoughts.

We radiate these waves around us all the time, and we attract the same kind of energy. This is why the people we live with or are in contact with the most become a part of our energy, waves, and behaviour. And when we choose to change our thoughts, patterns, and behaviour, we feel like we don't fit in anymore, and our social group also shows us that we're different.

That is why when you want to change something inside you or in your life, but you're unable to do it directly by changing your thoughts and patterns, changing your environment instead for the one you seek is a big step that can give you a fast result.

We first have to start with those that are closest to us—family. Our family gives us the base of our personality and most of our blueprints for many things: how we think about money, relationships, social conduct, etc. For the first seven years of our lives, we suck in everything presented to our senses—what we see, hear, touch, smell, taste, and feel (energy). As a baby, we're still open to the feeling of energy, until we lose it by not using it.

With that said, look back on all of the aspects of your life. Consider how your parents and siblings were doing and the life of your family at that time. It will tell you a lot about yourself!

After three years or so, we go to school, and there we enter the social world. There again, we're filled with information which makes us as we are now.

As a human, we desire to evolve, even if that desire is unconscious. We try to go beyond the rules we live in because nature is like that. To survive and grow, we need to expand our boundaries.

As conscious spiritual beings, we need to grow and continuously create new, better, and closer lives to the source of our being by becoming one with all energy. Our family gives us fertile ground for the start of our journey, and even if for some this ground is poor in nourishment for your mind, spirit or body, your need to grow will push you to search for a better way to be.

The trouble with that is that we create a powerful bond with our family. Emotionally, we get stuck to them in a way that makes it difficult for us to grow and go our way if we're not in a supportive, open-hearted, and loving family.

Our blood relations are, of course, important. They

provide a base to go to when we need it. Our family is a nest, where we should be safe and loved, whatever we do. I know that's not the case for everybody, and it's rather the opposite in many families. We often see our family as the cause of our present problems with ourselves, and we tend to reject them instead of understanding this gift.

I once eared that if we blame our parents for the bad in our lives, then we should also blame them for the good they gave us. For example, if they have been hard on you, it may make you want to be soft and kind.

Always look for the positive in all situations.

It can be challenging to maintain a healthy relationship with your family members when you think and act differently than they do. I had this kind of problem with my family due to my beliefs, diet, and success in life. My father felt that I was strange and took me off his life insurance so that I wouldn't get the money to pay for his funeral. He put only my sister on the policy. He based his decision only on the fact that I was different from him, that I had different beliefs, because financially I was doing better than my three sisters.

In order to grow and be ourselves, we need to move towards what we want to be. We need to be surrounded by the people we want to be like—not exactly like, but with the same status, happiness, and wealth in their relationships and environment. If you're going to become a Tibetan Buddhist monk, for example, then go and learn from them.

When you realize that you want to be something your family is absolutely not, and it blocks your growth, you need to take some distance from them. Not in your heart and relationship with them, but physically. Visit them less often or call them less. Reduce your contact, but keep the love and the connection alive when you are with them. Sometimes they might reject you, but that's their choice. Never let someone, even if it is your family, keep you from living your life and dreams. On this subject, family is a difficult topic.

Don't judge or blame yourself for having the desire to grow and be a better you.

Connect to what you desire. When you have a vision, personal or professional, find people who've achieved this same status already, as previously described. A happy father, a successful mom, a great speaker or teacher. Such a person doesn't need to be a billionaire near the end of their life, even though that person would certainly have a lot to teach you. I want to make clear that everybody can find a role model for every aspect of their lives.

It's step by step that we go further, and of course, some people can make you take giant steps, and if you can find one of those people, grab them and open your heart! But to be realistic, that kind of person is rare because they know the value of time and give it for a high price, or give it only to a few!

We are surrounded by people who have achieved at a level higher than us in all aspects of life. Search them out and find them, and when their level is no longer enough to help you grow, find another mentor or coach.

The same goes for your friends and colleagues. Who are your friends? Which aspects of their lives do you want to make better in your own? They're certainly equal to you. Here again, grow your circle of friends. Continue to see your actual friends, and at the same time, connect to new ones who have achieved what you want to achieve!

It's the same thing for what you want materially. Whether it's a car or a home, even if you can't afford it now, look at it, test drive that car, look at magazines about homes or vehicles that you desire, visit a home for sale to feel it and be there in person. Immerse yourself in the energy of what you want to accomplish or want to have, and feel it. Let the energy of it influence your energy, and let it become a part of you. Connect to it and grow the same energy in yourself, and it will be drawn to you. Of course, you need to use the three points detailed in Chapter 4, Power of Creation.

CHAPTER 7

POWER OF LEARNING
Educate Yourself

These days the schooling system may not be the best everywhere in the world. Some countries do better than others, but in the end, many students graduate with a lot of knowledge that they won't use in their lives. Worse still, they lack important fundamental knowledge, like how to do your taxes or how to be well connected to ourselves and the world around us (not digitally), and most important, how to use the knowledge that we have learned.

Formal education is not what will make us succeed at finding a way to be happy and fulfilled in our lives. By educating ourselves further, we will find a way.

We don't have any excuse for not doing it!

It is essential to educate ourselves in the subjects we love and need in order to experience growth in all aspects of our lives. We can learn anything if we are interested enough or in need of it.

Maybe you won't become an expert in every area, but learning will always give you benefits in your knowledge and abilities. To educate yourself is always a win.

And of course, please know that if you've read this far in this book, I'm so proud of you!

What are the essential areas to educate ourselves?

How does the mind work?

How does the body work?

How does our energetic being work?

Learn how to communicate with others and yourself.

Learn new skills, a sport, or a manual job.

Learn to play an instrument.

Learn a new way to do your job.

Whatever it is, everything is possible and infinite.

Let's hear an example with the story of a great publisher and businessman.

Let's call him Bob. Before finishing school, Bob had been kicked out and never went to college.

His teacher told him that he was stupid. But Bob thought differently.

After various events, Bob met a person who showed him the choices he had and showed him that he could do better. Bob had been learning what he wanted and putting it into practice.

Now he is the owner of an international publishing company that earns millions of dollars each year. All of that without a diploma!

If you search and research, you will find a lot of people who've achieved great success and have no diplomas, or who succeed in something different than what they studied.

This is to show you that everything is possible, even if you think you don't have the knowledge or the required diplomas.

Here's one other example: a 15-year-old boy who hates school but is very smart and has an excellent memory. But because he dislikes school, he doesn't do well there, and the teacher doesn't help him or like him.

However, in the subjects he likes, he has excellent grades, and in his hobbies, he can memorize huge amounts of information. He also has some real wisdom in him, and sometimes makes people feel amazed at what he says.

The problem with him is the lack of an enjoyable time in school. The rejection of some teachers doesn't make him feel good enough, even if he has great capacity. He will need to regain his self-confidence to see this about himself, and then he'll succeed in everything he wants, because with the enthusiasm he has, he will learn quickly.

Albert Einstein wrote, "Everybody is a genius. But if you judge a fish by its ability to climb a tree, it will live its whole life believing that it is stupid."

The question I have for you at this point of our journey together is "What is your talent?" Never doubt your capacity!

Read this repeatedly until you believe it: *I am smart enough to be capable of anything.*

Again, imagine yourself doing what you think you cannot do now. See yourself succeeding on your next test in school or playing the instrument you want. See yourself at your next job, which requires more knowledge than you have now, then *go learn that knowledge!*

A long time ago, I saw myself speaking to a large audience in a different language when I did not speak anything other than French.

Today, it's a reality! I could write for pages and pages about why we have to educate ourselves, but it's not necessary. Reread this if you need to process it and take it in.

Look around you to find more examples of people who don't have diplomas and still succeed in areas where we all think we cannot do without one.

CHAPTER 8

POWER OF NUTRITION

How to Eat Consciously

Before starting this subject, I want to notify you that nutrition is not the only factor for good health, and not the primary one either.

This is a significant and sensitive subject, hahaha!

I'm laughing already because I've had some sensitive discussions with my ex-wife about this. For many women on their period, churros are in their dreams, deep-fried dough covered in chocolate! I like them too, but only from my favourite place in Spain.

When it comes to our consciousness about food, body, energy, and belief, we all eat and enjoy at a different level.

To start with, know that what you eat now aligns

with your knowledge about food, health, and con-sciousness. And that is OK! There's no judgment implied from me, and most importantly, don't judge yourself!

We *all* have a history attached to what we eat, the meals we got from our parents, grandparents, and family as a child. For most of us, those meals shape our way of eating now.

Food itself can create addiction of a kind. Marketing also influences what we eat, as does our connection to nature.

Let me tell you about my journey with food; I share this with you to give you some idea of the processes that take place when we start to look at our eating habits. It is my path, and everyone has their own per-sonal way.

My father was a retired baker, and this was really nice for me. My memories are full of those weekends where I awoke to the smell of fresh bread, croissants, and pie. Mmm, I still drool from it.

I grew up with many bakeries around, and a tra-ditional meal was made of potatoes, rice or pasta, meat, and veggies. My father was a great cook, and I have been lucky to learn to eat many different things. I remember that I did have difficulties eating my piece of meat at a certain point, and I could not swallow it.

It caused me some trouble with my father, and meant chewing for a long time. I did grow up as a meat eater and did enjoy it for a long time.

When I started to develop my mind and spirituality, I looked at the effect of food on my physical body and my energy (the vibrations of cells, atoms, and also spiritual effects).

Along my journey in those areas, my way of looking at the food I was putting in my mouth changed without my thinking about it, and I started to eat differently. Not only what I was eating but *how* I was eating changed too!

The following is based on the perspective that a body can be healthy, energetic, and be in perfect balance with its environment.

OK, we'll get to the core of it now.

We eat from and for three different points.

First, to nourish our body.

The second is to nourish our emotions.

The third is to nourish our energy.

We all eat from those three points at different periods and frequencies.

Eating to nourish our body

We eat for the nourishment of the body. We need to eat for the survival of the body, and depending on where we are in the world, our climate influences what our body needs to stay alive. Living in the tropics doesn't require as many calories as living in the arctic circle. And here, pay attention; I say calories, not nutrients.

Calories are the fuel, and nutrients give the cells all the components for their most efficient activity.

In nature, all food is perfectly designed to be eaten by the right animal, human, bacteria, etc. As humans, we can eat and process almost every kind of edible food, from the heaviest food to the lightest and most easily digestible.

All-natural food will give us all the energy and nutrients for our body to live, be able to regenerate itself, and grow a solid immune system. Their energy (vibration) is also higher and brings us to a higher vibration level, supporting life.

We are a part of nature, and this magnificent body of ours is made from all the same elements that are found in nature. By eating what nature offers in its natural form, we support the life and structure of the body.

When we start to eat more food that is not directly from nature, or even fruits or veggies that are picked at an early stage and not ripe yet, we lose a big portion of the nutrients in those foods. For example, some berries produce enzymes recognized as natural cancer protection on their last days ripening on the bush.

This will affect our health in some ways because of the lack of freshness and life (vibration) in the food.

Cooking vegetables also affects their nutrients. This also contributes to a lack of nutrition, and with time, reduces our health and lifespan![2] The vibration is also reduced and changed.

Then, we might also eat 'dead food', which is any food that begins the rotting process directly as soon as we pick or kill it and needs to be processed directly to be conserved.

Most fruit and veggies continue their ripening process for a few days or even weeks after being harvested and stay alive until they start the rotting process, days or weeks after being picked.

When we eat this type of food, it is not only that

---

2.   Onyeka, Uloma and Ibeawchi, Obinna. "Loss of Food Nutrients orchestrated by Cooking Pots: a common trend in developing world." Published online by Cambridge University Press, 10 June 2020. https://www.cambridge.org/core/journals/proceedings-of-the-nutrition-society/article/loss-of-food-nutrients-orchestrated-by-cooking-pots-a-common-trend-in-developing-world/B9679B29E93E67E1C9DCCEF420413068

we lose out on a nutrient level, but also the vibration level of the food is lower and influences our body in its vibrational state.

The body, even if it can digest this food, will have more difficulty doing so and will use a significant amount of energy (calories) in this process.

This process also creates a more significant amount of waste to be disposed of, or that gets stuck in various parts of our body. In the process of digestion, the body also has to produce enzymes that put our health in a lower state.

And lastly, and certainly the most unhealthy, is all processed food packaged in cans or plastic and made from products that we don't know the origin of. This also includes the chemical products added to preserve food, such as adding red colour to meat when it is brown and less attractive. (In some places, such as Sweden, no colorant is added to the meat sold in supermarkets.)

All the products we put in processed food are unhealthy and come from chemical production.

Little is said about these products' negative effect on our health and mind, but nothing is done to ban or reduce them, or to educate people about them.

Besides its effect on our teeth, processed sugar is 1,000 times more addictive than cocaine! On a brain scan, we can see that cocaine lights up a tiny part of the brain, but sugar lights up a full party in the entire brain! Why? Because the brain is the primary consumer of sugar in the body.

Then, why do you find sugar in most processed foods in your supermarket? It makes you want to eat more of it and buy more of it also!

Cancer cells are also a great consumer of sugar. If you have cancer, help yourself by stopping a hundred percent of your consumption of processed sugar! (This is a bit of personal advice, not medical advice.)

Another product to consider is milk.

I will not speak much about it, and I advise you to educate yourself on this product. The only thing I can point you to is to ask why all animals in nature drink their mother's milk. Why do they all stop drinking it when they can start to eat by themselves and never return to drinking milk?

The next thing I want to share is this statistic about osteoporosis. The Nordic countries are the most significant consumers of dairy products and have the most osteoporosis cases.[3]

---

3. Karl Michaëlsson et al: "Milk intake and risk of mortality and fractures in women and men: cohort studies." *The BMJ*, October 2014. doi: https://doi. org/10.1136/bmj.g6015. 

I will not go further on that. I think it is essential that everyone go with their own knowledge and awareness to look into this and research the other products we put in our food.

Eating to nourish our social needs

Today, I think that most people in our modern society eat from this need. We don't think about why we eat; we feel hungry, and we choose the food that feels tasty and makes us feel good for the time we're eating it. And of course, most of the food that gives a warm feeling is processed and rich in fat, sugar, and other addictive and unhealthy substances.

Why do we always say what tastes good isn't healthy?

Let us look at this closely. Psychologically, we have been wired to connect food and emotion since we were babies. When a baby is hungry, it cries, and then it gets to drink from the breast of its mother, in a natural world. What is more comforting than that? I'm a man, and I still like the breast of a woman!

Seriously though, food brings us comfort from the time we are babies, and our education about nutrition teaches us that food is comforting for us.

For me as a child, a good apple pie made by my

father brought comfort and a sense of the feast we had on the weekends when my father baked, and we did eat pie, excellent bread, and other delicious delicacies.

Food is comforting when we feel sad and alone. Food fills up our belly, the centre of our emotions, and makes us feel full when our mind and soul feel empty and lonely.

Food brings us memories of a past time, and is why we go back to some meals we used to eat as a child. And of course, we complain that the meal doesn't taste the same as the one our grandmothers made!

For many people who desire to lose weight and fail at it, it's not because they aren't determined or focused enough, but simply because the problem lies on a psychological and emotional level.

We have a lot of different psychological and emotional reasons for eating comforting food, and it's our job to examine them for our own good.

It's pretty easy to understand and to work on it. When you want to eat something, ask yourself these simple questions.

What do I feel now? What is my emotional state?

For which kind of food am I hungry now?

When was the last time I ate?

Tell yourself to take a piece of fruit or another natural, healthy food and see how you feel about it. Those questions are put in random order, and can be used in any order you like. One can lead you to another.

Here I will give a little example for each question to make it easy to understand and see what they can provide you.

First: What do I feel? What is my emotional state?

This question will make you focus for a moment on yourself and allow you to recognize your feelings and emotional state at the moment. It will also allow you to see that what you feel is not hunger but emptiness or sadness that you try to suppress.

The other benefit to this question is to give you the possibility to change your emotional state. Get in control of your emotions and don't be owned by them—instead, own them. Eating to suppress emotion doesn't serve us. It makes us sick. Recognizing all our feelings allows us to transform them and let them pass.

Second question: For which kind of food am I hungry now?

This question will give you a good indication of why you are hungry. It can be because of some real hunger; maybe you did not eat for the last day, or your body asks you for real nutrition and makes you crave a particular fruit or veggie, or water. Or, like the example above, it may be to comfort some emotional state.

The third question is related to the second: When was the last time I ate?

When did you eat a good piece of healthy fruit? Again, you may crave anything just because you feel like you need to get energy after a long day of hard work.

You want yourself to grab some fruit, but you feel like, "No, I prefer this bag of chips." This can give you also some good indication of why you want to eat and what.

By asking those questions every time you want to eat, you will gain awareness within yourself about your eating habits and emotional state.

This awareness leads you on a particularly good path to creating a better emotional and physical environment for yourself, along with using the information in this book and all you will learn by yourself.

As social animals, we also eat for a social factor.

All the different celebrations in diverse cultures and countries are occasions to get together and share a meal.

During those events, we can feel forced in some ways to eat what we don't normally eat, or eat too much most of the time. It can be challenging for those who don't eat the same way as their family or friends to get involved in some of those social gatherings, especially if they judge your food habits or think that you cannot participate because they eat what you don't. It is a social issue that can separate people.

For example, when I stopped eating meat, my sister stopped inviting me for supper and some barbecues because she thought she could not provide anything for me. I had to explain to her that not having meat was not a problem and a good salad with potatoes cooked on the barbecue was also really good for me. Without announcing it, I brought some preparations of my own, which made everybody drool over my plate.

Whatever your differences, don't let them be a separation factor in your life.

Eating to nourish our energy

This section is about the interaction of the vibrations of our food and the vibrations of our body.

First, a little bit of science. Everything living in nature is made of molecules, which are themselves made of atoms. The atoms are made of smaller particles, and finally, we can now see that those smaller particles are made of energy—of vibrations.

In our body, we have about 37 trillion cells, more or less, all made of atoms. Each of them is vibrating, and we can locally or globally read the level of vibration of the human body or each organ by example.

The same applies for an apple, or broccoli, water, a steak, or a glass of wine. Like radio waves can be tuned to capture a radio station, those same waves can be broadcast to an tomato and we can see its effect.[4]

The result is that by applying a different frequency level, we can modify the tomato, which leads us to our topic: eating to nourish our energy.

Some research shows that a healthy body has a high vibration level.[5]

We use the expression "Wow, you look vibrant," because a high vibration level is the expression of life. A cell in our body that stops vibrating is dead. And a low level of vibration is an open door for sickness.

The food we eat has the same effect on our cells as the radio waves put into the tomato in the experiment.

---

4.   Altunas, Ozlem and Ozkurt, Halil. "The assessment of tomato fruit quality parameters under different sound waves." *Journal of Food Science and Technology*, 2019 Apr; 56(4): 2186–2194. https://www.ncbi.nlm.nih.gov/pmc/articles/PMC6443699.

5.   Schomburg, Tina. "How to Heal Your Body by Using the Frequency of Life." Oct. 23, 2014. https://medium.com/meducated-org/how-to-heal-your-body-by-using-the-frequency-of-life-9307af550fbb

With its own vibration level, the tomato influences our vibration.

When we can understand this physical process, we can see the relationship between living food and dead food within our level of energy and health.

Again, see this as informative and not meant as judgment. Ultimately, there isn't a good way to eat or a bad one; there are only different ways that take us on different paths.

What are the effects of eating to increase our energy or reduce it?

One of the most obvious is to our health. Of course, many of us have had the experience eating a good, warm heavy meal, full of cooked, processed food that's also in the rotting process. (See the definition of 'dead food' in the first part of this chapter.)

Then we feel heavy, full, and sleepy with no energy.

And in the opposite case, we all have had the experience of eating some colourful salad in the summertime, full of fresh veggies and fruit that left us feeling full of energy, fully awake, and with more clarity of thought.

Like I described in the first part of this chapter, food has its own energy and the farther we take it from its natural form and process it, or if we eat it when it's in its rotting process, the more its energy (level of vibration) is lowered. Its effect on our cells makes our vibration level go up or down. It can lead our body to better health or diminishes our health.

One other effect of food is on our ability to think clearly. When the level of vibration of our body is rising, all our systems work more efficiently, and it brings us more clarity in our thoughts and feelings. Connection in the energy feels clearer and accessible. That can also give us a better understanding and sense of intuition.

When your whole body is vibrating at a higher level of energy, you also influence everything around you and whatever you are in tune with.

If you attune yourself with a healthy, high-vibrating body, you will attract more of this energy (law of attraction). You will experience more feelings of energy and health in your life. You will be able to do more, be less tired, have more ideas, and have more mental clarity.

Conversely, by eating food with a lower level of energy, you will have less energy and less clarity of thought, and then you may experience more trouble in your emotions and health. It will tune you in with the same energy you broadcast and make you experience lower energy and health.

But food is not the only factor that influences your physical and emotional health. Your state of mind also influences you at a great level!

We modern humans live in a world that gives us everything on a plate—literally. Many people don't know where their food comes from, how it's grown or made, or what's inside it.

For example, a study in Britain showed that kids did not know where the milk they were drinking came from. The most common answer was "from the supermarket."[6]

One of my own studies showed me that people of different ages think that meat is different from the muscle of the animal they eat. It's something I have to admit made me think, "Well, what do they think they're eating then?"

This is why I want to offer you this little meditation. The first attempt may take a bit of time, but if you choose to do it regularly, you can do it at the speed of your thoughts.

Eating in consciousness

For this example, we will take an orange.

Sit at your table, or wherever you want, and peel

---

6.   "Survey shows a third of British children don't know where milk comes from." *Farming UK*, 28 June 2017. https://www.farminguk.com/news/ survey-shows-a-third-of-british-children-don-t- know-where-milk-comes-from_46824.html

an orange. Eat part of it and keep the rest. Now, close your eyes and imagine a seed of the orange in the beautiful, dark earth. The seed is covered in the dark, and slowly a sprout grows out of it!

With a lot of force and determination, the sprout grows upward and reaches the surface of the ground. There, it starts to feel the sun and grow into a little tree. The sun, the rain, and the wind given to this tree made it grow, and now after a long and patient process, it becomes an enormous tree.

The tree shares her beautiful flowers for us to see and for the bees to eat. You can see a small orange starting to grow and grow from one flower. It eats the sun and drinks the water.

Now the orange is ripe, and a hand comes to pick it. She is a worker, a woman, and by working in the orchard, she can feed her family and be happy. This orange passes from the orchard to a truck and onto a plane and arrives in your country. It is transported to your supermarket, and there you pick it up.

At this point, this orange has given work and joy to many people. Now you bring it home, and you just peel it. It's time to eat one other piece. Eat it and see for yourself if you taste it differently than the first piece.

Do you feel differently about the orange? See for yourself, and now as quick as you think your thoughts, you can do that for all the food you eat. You can think about the life of the food you will eat, what work has been put in during the process of getting that food to you, the lives that have been touched by it, and all you can imagine. Now, I will let you enjoy your next meal.

POWER OF ANCIENT TRADITION, POWER OF NATURE

Now that we have made some ground, I would like to introduce you to the power of nature and her elements. We physically belong to the earth, and are made of all the same elements.

Ancient traditions all around the globe use the same elements to have access to greater knowledge, and as a healing process for the emotional and spiritual aspects of our life. Here, I would like to address two of them: the fire walk, and the sweat lodge.

The fire walk

The fire walk is a tradition in which we use the energy of fire for transformation, like the phoenix reborn from its ashes!

We transform, and not only by walking on glowing, burning coals in this ceremony. It is during the entire process of building the wood fire, lighting it, and watching it burn that we go and connect to the energy of fire and our intention. By focusing on what we want to transform, we light the fire within ourselves.

Fire has the power to transform; it transmutes solid elements into pure energy and allows life to prosper. Its energy has the same effect on us; it transforms and enables us to grow anew within.

Fire is life in action. Don't we say, "Wow, I am on fire today," when we have a lot of energy and succeed at what we're doing? Fire is what we feel when we experience any emotion to an extreme. We start to feel physically warm.

Fire moves things around it. It moves molecules just as it moves our energy.

I can't write too much about it, because it's an experience that everyone who wants to has to feel for themselves, and no two experiences will be alike.

From my own experience, I can say that it's

important who leads you through the process. Always trust your intuition when you pick somebody to direct a fire walk.

The sweat lodge

The ceremony of the sweat lodge symbolizes birth and rebirth. The sweat lodge represents the womb of Mother Earth.

As a part of the ceremony, fire is used to heat stones to a red glowing point, which are then taken inside the sweat lodge and sprayed with water. It creates a warm, humid environment within the sweat lodge, like a womb. Except for the glowing stones, it's dark inside.

Here again, the fire brings on transformation in combination with the water's energy of life. Water has a living emotional energy that's flowing and flexible. It moves deep within us, carries our emotions, and supports all life.

During a sweat lodge ceremony, we connect with the cardinal points and the energy connected to them. Each direction is related to an animal and its energy.

Again, the person who leads you in the process plays an essential role. There are many different traditions for the sweat lodge, and they are used for various purposes or intentions. The ceremony can be open to everyone, or only allow men or women. There may be only one opening or an opening for entering and exiting. It depends on the tradition of your country, the purpose for the ceremony, and the one leading it.

For me, it has been a unique experience each time I participated. Again, see and experience it for yourself.

Before introducing you to another aspect of self-development, I'd like you to think about what we value and how we value it when it comes to personal development. In all the workshops you may attend, whether it's a dancing soul meeting, a sweat lodge, or voice work, the price you pay will not influence the result. In some countries it's customary to ask for a lot of money for some of these workshops, leading some people to believe that the more you pay, the more you'll get out of them. We have to create our own wealth, even if we do good for the world. I also understand the need to be well paid for the time we offer. At the same time, it's important for you to know how much you need to pay to feel that what you're learning has real value and real quality. We can give some people free sessions of coaching or energy healing because giving is the secret to happiness. Meanwhile, clients are willing to pay for the same service because for them, the service they get is worth the price.

Everyone's financial state is different, as are their thoughts about how much they can invest in themselves. In my case, I learned that we are priceless, and we don't need to be cheap with ourselves. At the same time, we can't be stupid either.

Energy healing

Now, I'd like to ask you to open your field of possibilities even more and introduce you to the opportunity to use energy to help yourself.

As we've seen, everything in us is made of energy. Our thoughts are energy, and our focus moves it. Now imagine using this energy to heal yourself at a different level of being and intensity.

Ancient traditions around the world have used energy for healing for centuries. They call the energy *chi* in Asia, other places call it magnetism, and still many other names are used in different traditions and parts of the world. Energy healing techniques such as Reiki and others have been brought to the West from Eastern countries. We can find healers who work with the power of thought and energy in all countries and traditions.

Imagine doing it yourself now. The ability to do so comes with an understanding of who you are, a belief in your ability to use and move the energy, and knowing that you create your reality with the projection of your thoughts.

You can start to play with the energy of your body by feeling it between your hands, and through meditation, make it move and feel it in your body. You can learn from masters in different arts, such as the *chi gong* or *tai chi chuan.*

You can educate yourself on this topic to find out more information and get what you need to receive from it. Follow your intuition and let all possibilities exist.

Afterword

would like to go deeper with our role as creators of our reality. For many years, I knew that all my thoughts, words, and actions created my reality and the world I live in. But it was only a piece of knowledge to me—I saw it and learned it, but at the same time, it was still a kind of external knowledge.

Until one day, I was walking in the forest and talking to myself and from nowhere this *aha!* moment happened. I felt deep within me a feeling of realization, of integration about this knowledge I have. It became an experience and something true for me.

We are the co-creator of our reality. We co-create all on Earth, using the greatest energy, which also created us. We are more powerful than we can believe, we are more beautiful than how we see ourselves, and we are more loved than we think. We are more connected to the rest of the world, to all humans, animals, and plants, than we think.

The world has been a rough place for a long time, and the illusion of separation has created all the horror we see around us, but this is only because we have forgotten who we are and what we can do—what is our real power within.

By learning more about ourselves, being more conscious of our connection to all life, knowing and using our capacity to co-create the world we want to live in, and taking responsibility, we can unleash the power within us. It's this exact same power that we have been created from.

We are limitless in all aspects of our lives. In creating more separation or connection, we can choose to create at a fantastic scale whatever we want.

In my case, I desire more love and harmony for all of us, and I know we are all connected to our source. In each one of you reading this page now glows beautiful energy of love and light. Now, we are connected as you touch and read those lines Your thought is directed to me and mine to you as I write this.

You are beautiful, loved, and amazing beyond measure. I love you for who you are. Love your magnificent self, and you will love all.

www.ingramcontent.com/pod-product-compliance
Lightning Source LLC
Chambersburg PA
CBHW052056150726
48002CB00002B/910